**Transforming Healthcare**

# Transforming Healthcare

An Insider's Look on Why and How

*Morey Menacker*

**JB** JOSSEY-BASS™
A Wiley Brand

Published by John Wiley & Sons, Inc., Hoboken, New Jersey.
Published simultaneously in Canada.

For general information on our other products and services or for technical support, please contact our Customer Care Department within the United States at (800) 762-2974, outside the United States at (317) 572-3993 or fax (317) 572-4002.

Wiley also publishes its books in a variety of electronic formats. Some content that appears in print may not be available in electronic formats. For more information about Wiley products, visit our web site at www.wiley.com.

*Library of Congress Cataloging-in-Publication Data applied for:*

Paperback: 9781119902522

Cover Design: Wiley
Cover Image: © leowolfert/Adobe Stock Photos

Set in 9.5/12.5pt STIXTwoText by Straive, Chennai, India

SKY10034665_061322

# Contents

# Contents

# Foreword

I have had the past good fortune on several occasions of meeting certain persons for the first time, who, after hearing them speak cogently for only a few minutes, have become my instant and durable friends. One such colleague is Dr. Morey Menacker, former President and Chief Executive Officer of the highly successful New Jersey-based Hackensack Alliance Accountable Care Organization, and well qualified author of this brave new book, *Transforming Healthcare*. Given his very extensive experience as a master geriatrician and seasoned senior healthcare executive, the best three words I can think of to describe Morey are as "The Doctor's Doctor".

More than twenty years ago, the Institute of Medicine (now known as the National Academy of Medicine within the National Academy of Sciences) published an urgent "call to action" for the American Health System in its seminal *Crossing the Quality Chasm*. This consensus-based work defined quality of healthcare through six very important aims: Care that is simultaneously Safe, Timely, Efficient, Effective, Equitable and Patient-Centered. In this regard, *Transforming Healthcare* continues to fire on all of these cylinders as the vision of the future is presented.

One of these aims is "Efficiency", which the IOM originally defined as "avoiding waste, including waste of equipment, supplies, ideas, and energy". I emphasize this definition often when discussing the time-honored topic of "Cost of Care", because it helps gets at heart of the economic mindset that is necessary for realizing what's at stake throughout this book. Yet, today's determinations as to what constitutes optimally efficient healthcare depends on which lens the many diverse stakeholders among the US healthcare system use for their own internal deliberations. And, as Dr. Menacker rightly points out, major challenges to overcome this resultant inertia stand in the way to achieving timely consensus-based solutions for improved health status, such as redirecting resources towards improved patient-centered primordial prevention efforts and away from our traditional delivery of downstream "sickness treatment". Yet, at the end of 2021, the market cap of the healthcare industry exceeds $5 Trillion and per capita healthcare costs total $4.5 Trillion. Unfortunately, the Cost Curve is bending in the wrong direction, i.e. concave up, not convex down.

An important and illustrative example to denote in the context of *Transforming Healthcare* is cardiovascular disease (CVD), which is the leading cause of death, not only in the US, but for the entire world. CVD (including acute myocardial infarction, heart failure and other patients with coronary atherosclerosis), when combined with stroke account for four of the top 10 expensive conditions treated annually in US hospitals. Most major local and regional US hospitals provide comprehensive acute care services to patients with major acute cardiovascular events (MACE), including well-staffed medical and surgical intensive care units, sophisticated state-of-the art technologies and procedure rooms for acute high-definition imaging and multimodal revascularization interventions, and specialist physicians, nurses, pharmacists and other healthcare professionals with advanced training credentials. Well paid and incentivized traditional health system service line senior executives skillfully juggle day-to-day operations, complex and interdependent supply chains, ever-evolving information technologies, challenging workforce requirements, managed care negotiations and increasing capital allocations. Chief Executive Officers and their governing boards prioritize the "strategic" intention of these service lines in order to realize substantial future revenue growth through increased market share and reimbursement and competitive advantage for being recognized regionally as "cutting edge and ahead of the curve".

In contrast, High Blood Pressure (HBP), a major risk factor for MACE, results in billions of dollars of waste from reduced worker productivity and absenteeism as well as significant increased per capita healthcare costs. Clearly, reducing the risk of major cardiovascular events by controlling HBP, and thereby improving health-related quality of life, can significantly lower attributable excess annual per capita health costs. High quality scientific evidence from large scale population-based studies published in the 2017 Hypertension Clinical Practice Guidelines of the American Heart Association (AHA) and the American College of Cardiology (ACC) documents the significant blood pressure lowering effects from six specific critically important lifestyle modifications: tobacco cessation, regular physical exercise, restriction of dietary sodium, dietary intake of potassium, moderate alcohol consumption and a "healthy heart" diet. Assessments of Social Determinants of Health (SDoH), Shared Decision Making (SDM) conversations between patients and their physicians, and Team-Based Care (TBC) delivered by nurses, pharmacists and other health professionals are now known to result in significant improvement in BP control and other health risk reduction targets through effective, evidence-based lifestyle modifications.

Nonetheless, recent data reveals that over 115 million Americans have diagnosed or undiagnosed HBP, and that more than half are inadequately controlled to guideline-based BP targets published by AHA and ACC. Worst of all, blood pressure is almost always measured incorrectly, resulting in innumerable inaccurate readings obtained in both health care settings and at home. Inadequately controlled HBP is but one of many major unmet public health challenges that can be directly traced to the diffuse health system inertia so elegantly addressed by Dr. Menacker in Chapter 5 of *Transforming Healthcare* that is at the heart of this matter. No doubt, the healthcare delivery infrastructure for the care of major acute and chronic CVD is vastly different than what is needed to achieve health promotion, maintenance, and prevention necessary to reduce MACE and hence the need for acute care.

I recently asked some health system senior managers, governing board members and primary care physicians to informally describe the barriers to achieving optimal BP control. Their comments were remarkably consistent and focused on time and resource constraints, process limitations and a general lack of urgency regarding HBP as a top organizational priority. The clinicians described control of HBP as "just another metric" within constantly expanding externally imposed quality requirements. Administrative demands remain overly burdensome, leading to too many "clicks" to add home BP readings to the electronic health record (EHR). In addition, the team is understaffed and overworked, leaving no time to properly address Social Determinants of Health (SDoH) and effective lifestyle modifications. Traditional practices do not ensure consistent and accurate BP measurement technique with validated and certified devices in accordance with standardized guideline-based scientific methods. Patients often present other pressing concerns, which can lead to deferment of BP control until the next annual examination or ignoring it altogether. Not surprisingly, control of HBP for patients and employees is nowhere to be found as a key performance indicator on any governance or managerial accountability "dashboards".

Of course, it is certainly much easier for us to describe these "wicked" problems like control of HBP than to find and implement cogently clear pathways to solving them. And while Dr. Menacker's strong recommendation for global payments to health systems to simultaneously manage the associated clinical and financial risks is not new, it comes at just the right time in our history. What is urgently needed today to achieve the goals outlined in this book are stronger health system alliances and congruent alignment with insurers, employers, public health, community health safety net organizations, large and small biopharmaceutical and device firms, digital health Information technology companies and governmental health agencies. "Moving the Needle" of improved health status of the US population will require a major reprioritization of both capital and human resource allocation by all of these stakeholders. *Transforming Healthcare* is henceforth our Call to Action.

Principal & Founder, IPO 4 Health (Improving Patient Outcomes 4 Health)
Associate Professor of Medicine, Rush Medical College
Senior Associate Editor,
American Journal of Medical Quality  *Donald E. Casey Jr*
*MD, MPH, MBA, FACP,*
*FAHA, CPE, DFAAPL, DFACMQ*

## About the Companion Website

This book is accompanied by a companion website.

**www.wiley.com/go/menacker/transforminghealthcare**

This website includes:

- Test Banks
- PowerPoint Lecture Slides

# Introduction

One may ask, "Why would a physician who has worked for years in our current healthcare system want to transform said system?" While there is no easy answer, I will try to explain. My postgraduate training took place in an inner city environment, where the majority of patients were hospitalized due to complications of their environment. This included drug addiction, poorly controlled hypertension, diabetes, hyperlipidemia, food insecurity, homelessness, and trauma. It became obvious early in my career that prevention was infinitely cheaper, and more rewarding, than treatment. The conundrum was in developing a method to pay for prevention.

It is imperative that those of us who work in a particular field, and benefit financially from that work, must give back in some way as gratitude for the opportunity, and to preserve these opportunities for future generations. It is also much easier to comment and suggest change in a field that has defined your entire life. We all have a responsibility to leave this world a better place than we found it.

It is common occurrence that when an international celebrity, or a wealthy foreigner, becomes ill, they automatically fly to the United States for their healthcare. These individuals would not come here if they thought the medical care was inferior. However, we are constantly bombarded by the media with tales of inadequate care, greed, malpractice, and refusal to provide needed services. Is it possible for these two disparate stories to both be true? The answer is a resounding YES. We are blessed with the best technology, the best treatments, the best research, the best hospitals, and the best physicians, yet the care provided can be disjointed, inadequate at times, cost prohibitive, and occasionally inappropriate.

This book attempts to explain how we got to this place and how we can get better.

# 1

# How Did We Get Here?

A common theme at healthcare conferences, in blogs, journals, and books is the topic of problems with the US healthcare system. This topic is prominent because the current refrain is that "healthcare is broken." There are many examples offered, including: lack of access to care, cost of insurance and medications, rising percent of GDP (Gross Domestic Product) consumed by healthcare, infant mortality rates, rural hospital closures, physician shortage, nursing shortage, and the uninsured. Many solutions are also offered, including: single payer system (Medicare for All), Obamacare 2.0, legislating pricing controls, healthcare *disruptors*, elimination of medical school tuition, and others. A common argument includes the caveat to keep what's good, but change what's bad. In other words, "let me keep my health insurance, fix the system, but don't ask me to change, because I like what I have."

In order to understand how we got to this point, a little historical perspective is helpful. The concept of health insurance coincided with the birth of unions, early in the twentieth century. Many unions requested medical care for their injured workers and this slowly expanded to comprehensive medical care for workers and their families. Following World War II, there was an attempt to nationalize healthcare by President Truman, which was unsuccessful. However, this effort eventually led to the enactment of Medicare, healthcare coverage for the elderly. In 1965, President Johnson signed the bill creating Medicare. Under the bill, anyone over the age of 65 would automatically receive coverage for Part A, which paid for 80% of hospitalization costs. Coverage for Part B, outpatient costs, was available with an additional attached. Commercial insurance at that time was also divided into hospitalization and

*Transforming Healthcare: An Insider's Look on Why and How*, First Edition. Morey Menacker.
© 2022 John Wiley & Sons, Inc. Published 2022 by John Wiley & Sons, Inc.
Companion website: www.wiley.com/go/menacker/transforminghealthcare

outpatient. At the time, physician office visits were affordable for most adults, but the concern was the rising cost of hospital stays. Secondary, or "gap" insurance was available for purchase, to cover the 20% not covered by Medicare. The Federal Government had no method of determining appropriate payment for healthcare services, so they borrowed from Blue Cross/Blue Shield the "reasonable and customary" approach to payment. Following treatment, a patient would receive a bill and be expected to pay. Medicare would determine what the "usual and customary" fee should be and reimbursed the patient at an 80% level. Any services provided in a hospital setting were billed individually. Many providers and hospitals recognized that they were able to set the "usual and customary" rate by routinely charging an inflated amount to all patients. That number would then become the "usual and customary" rate, even if the full amount was never received. The providers felt that if they received a portion of the inflated bill from a third-party source, either the government or a health insurance company, they could waive the patient's responsibility and everyone would be happy. These inflated bills were the first sign of the ever-increasing disparity between "healthcare charges" and "healthcare costs." This process continued unfettered until 1983 when the Prospective Payment System (PPS) was signed into law by President Reagan. In 1978, New Jersey embarked on a demonstration project that went live in 1980. Payments to hospitals would be bundled into a single payment. This payment would be calculated by the patient's diagnosis, not the charges generated for services performed. It was known as DRG payments, or Diagnosis Related Groups. This pertained only to the Medicare population, but many commercial insurers soon followed suit. As the Federal Government struggled with the rapid rise in healthcare spending, a decision was reached to expand the New Jersey initiative to the entire country. This was known as the Prospective Payment System (PPS), and moved all hospital billing for Medicare patients to DRG. An unintended consequence of the PPS was the need to provide inpatient services to patients not meeting criteria for acute hospitalization, therefore not meeting Medicare's criteria for payment. Prior to this legislation, patients could be admitted to the hospital for any reason, without question. Services were billed in an itemized fashion, including hotel services (the actual hospital stay, food service, housekeeping, etc.), procedures, diagnostics, medications, and other treatments. Professional services were billed independently. The introduction of DRG payments meant hospitals were paid for the patient's diagnosis and the shorter the stay, the greater potential for profit. However, many of these patients were not well enough to go home and care for themselves. This gave rise to the concept of Subacute Care, which would be paid by Medicare on a per diem basis, or daily rate. This was devised because a study performed at the time suggested that patients would only need a few days of subacute care following hospitalization. Initially, this care was provided in the hospital setting, separate and distinct from the DRG-based acute hospitalization. However, over time, the nursing home industry realized the potential windfall of third party funded, short-term stay, patient care opportunities; and criteria were developed to certify nursing homes as subacute care facilities. Authorization was required from Medicare to certify the need for subacute care. As the volume increased, and CMS (Center for Medicare/Medicaid Services) was unable to process these authorizations promptly, Medicare determined that the initial authorization would be acceptable for up to a 20 day stay. Rather than create a DRG system for subacute care, Medicare persisted in paying a daily rate to nursing homes, encouraging the facilities to keep all patients the maximum allowable days. Hospitals began to realize that they could transfer patients previously requiring acute care to the newly certified subacute facilities, and still receive the full DRG payment for the acute hospitalization. This created sicker patients entering subacute care, where the staffing was still at nursing home levels, and the skill level was marginal. Patients would show deteriorating health and be returned to the hospital, where a new DRG rate would be initiated. The attempt to stem the rising cost of hospital care actually caused a more rapid increase in healthcare spending, albeit unintentionally. More recently, CMS has tried to control this revolving door by decreasing payments for hospital readmissions within 30 days of discharge [1, 2].

The next significant change in Medicare payments came in 1992, when physician payments moved from "usual and customary" to RBRVS, the Resource-Based Relative Value Score. In 1988, an article was published in the *Journal of the American Medical Association* by Harvard researchers recommending this standardization for physician payment. RBRVS created a relative value to each procedure code available to physicians and this value was adjusted by region of the country. The payment had three factors: physician work, practice expense, and malpractice expense. This system, which was supposed to standardize physician payment, has multiple flaws. Most importantly, the value is skewed toward procedures that require physical skills, such as surgery and interventions. The value placed upon diagnostic skill is minimized and does not differentiate between treatment of a common cold versus diagnosing an uncommon disease that leads to a lifesaving treatment. In addition, the scale does not account for appropriateness or outcomes. Theoretically, a surgeon could be paid every single time he repairs the same hernia on a patient, even though his technique may have induced the recurrence, or even multiple recurrences. This payment model actually incentivizes overuse and more complicated procedures. In essence, the efforts to stem the rapid rise in healthcare spending, while reining in abuse of the system, has created new and inventive methods to increase Medicare spending without improving outcomes [3–6].

At the time of Medicare creation, the average mortality age in the United States was in the early seventies, so the expected length of services provided by Medicare was less than 10 years per person. Today, that length of services provided is doubled, due to a longer average lifespan. The number of Medicare beneficiaries has also expanded due to baby boomers aging. If our per-person spend per-year had remained stable, our total spend would have multiplied, due to increased patient years, and the larger number of beneficiaries. However, the annual Medicare budget has grown far beyond expectations, as healthcare spend per person has skyrocketed as well.

While it is true that, since the creation of Medicare, our ability to treat many diseases has improved, the driver of increased per person spending is not solely due to new treatments. The hospital business suddenly had a third party payer with deep pockets, the federal government, and the "big dogs" knew how to eat.

Early in the twentieth century, hospitals had very limited treatments available for patients. Other than surgery, there was not much done for patients. Birthing was still performed at home. Antibiotics were not readily available until World War II. Innovations in medical equipment occurred, but were cost prohibitive, as there was no organized financing (health insurance) to pay for hospital services. The development of Medicare, paired with tax deductible employer-sponsored health insurance, allowed hospitals to charge a third party for medical testing and treatment. In fact, the model developed where insurance (and Medicare) would pay a percentage of charges, NOT COSTS.

This was a goldmine, as hospitals (and doctors) could bill excessive charges, and cost shift for the care of the uninsured or underinsured. It also generated the capital investment for hospitals to enlarge and purchase more and more equipment and technology. It was all paid for! The sicker the patient, the higher the charge, and the higher the payment. We spend exorbitantly on treating the sick, but allocate almost no resources on good health. We allow neighboring hospitals to invest heavily in high-priced technology and treatments, causing them to compete for the same sick patients in order to pay for these upgrades. If the location where services were delivered was controlled, and efficiency was incumbent upon the providers of these services, we could dramatically cut spending. These dollars could go toward improving health, thereby decreasing further the need for expensive hospital services. While there are some guardrails currently in place to control runaway spending, hospitals continue to focus on the highest billable service, not necessarily the best outcome. A case in point is the use of robotic surgery to perform an appendectomy. An emergency appendectomy can be performed manually by a surgeon in under 30 minutes, and, if uncomplicated, the patient can go home the same day. Many hospitals encourage the surgeons to use a robot for this procedure. It commonly can lengthen the procedure fivefold, but can be billed (and paid) at a much higher rate. Outcomes are not improved, but pockets are fuller.

This example is only one of many affecting our ability to control healthcare spending. The concept of a cost-based pricing system is common to many areas of business in the United States. This system creates a price structure based on the cost of providing the service. In general, there is a small percentage added for profit. Hospitals work on a charge-based system, calculating a percentage of Medicare allowable charges and negotiation with health insurance companies. Most hospitals lose money on Medicare DRG payments, and either cost shift to commercial payers or cover their losses with inflated fees for outpatient care provided by the hospital. Almost any outpatient procedure performed at a hospital carries a higher charge than if performed at an independent outpatient facility. Whether the cost of this procedure is higher at a hospital is information no one has determined, or even asked. Health insurance companies negotiate rates with hospitals and providers based on local competition, patient preference, and volume. The motivation by the insurers is to drive as many patients as possible to purchase their plans, as their profits are driven solely by volume of beneficiaries. The insurance companies then calculate the cost of service and transfer the expense to the patient, via an increase in the insurance premium. There is no incentive to curb costs by either party. This has all been driven by lack of government oversight in the cost of care, quality of care, efficiency of care, and outcomes of care. Can we expect (or trust) the government to fix our "broken system?" The transformation required is to change the financing method, in order to incentivize patients and providers to keep everyone healthy. If we pay to treat illness, is it really in a healthcare provider's best interest to prevent disease? This is not unlike the auto industry's "built in obsolescence." If the auto industry produced a car that would run forever, people would stop buying new cars. Therefore, they must build cars with a limited lifespan.

The above examples of the broken healthcare system are all true. We have the ability to fix all of them. However, the solutions currently being offered will not fix the problems and there is no one solution for all the ills identified. This is where inertia comes in. We have a tendency to repeat the same actions, and change requires a certain amount of energy, or momentum. Whenever we strive for change, we must create energy, or momentum for change. This energy initiates the motion toward a new steady state and overcomes the inertia of the status quo. In order to achieve the desired effect, three questions must be answered: Why, What, and How. Why should we do this differently? What are we trying to accomplish? How do we do this?

Whenever we hear of plans to fix the broken healthcare system, we should ask those three questions. The answers do not exist within any of the current "solutions." Merely throwing money at a problem does not fix it. First, one must clearly identify the problem and then develop a coherent treatment plan. We talk about lack of access to care, but do not consider the ability to afford medications. If we tackle access and cost of medications, how do we ensure adherence to treatment? If we create a plan to improve adherence, can we guarantee adequate healthy food and shelter?

A common cry in response to these questions is "you are talking about Social Determinants of Health." Since when was this NOT part of healthcare? All of the countries providing universal healthcare also include significant social services for all, as part of the healthcare system. We spend much more money per person treating illnesses that are the effects of social inequality or a result of the lack of adequate food and shelter.

Most countries providing nationalized healthcare to their citizens also provide enhanced social services to those in need. These services prevent or minimize many problems that our country spends millions of dollars to treat. An example would be adequate prenatal care, nutrition, and vitamins for all pregnant women. This has been shown to dramatically decrease infant mortality and morbidity. Yet we choose to spend the money on premature infants and childhood illness. A much more efficient method would be to spend money on prevention. There was an old commercial on television about preventive car maintenance that had a slogan "you can pay me now, or pay me later." Since treatment of illness is a much more definable product, we are comfortable spending money "later," rather than a much smaller amount earlier on prevention [7, 8].

It is true that our country has a much more diverse population than many countries with nationalized healthcare, who tend to be smaller and more homogeneous. However, the argument here is not for nationalization of healthcare; it is for shifting our financial focus upstream, toward prevention. While most believe that this effort would require government oversight, our current system of healthcare financing already requires government oversight and monitoring. This type of reallocation already occurs in other domains, with federal subsidies for state managed Medicaid programs, public schools, and farmers. We could easily establish a plan to move healthcare dollars toward accepted preventive measures and social determinants, without creating a nationalized healthcare system [7, 8].

The single most effective healthcare innovation in the nineteenth century was the development of the London sewer system. More lives were saved by controlling sewage and allowing for clean drinking water than any other single discovery or invention. In the twentieth century, vaccination was the single most effective healthcare innovation. These innovations both were preventive in nature and saved millions of lives. Perhaps one solution to the current healthcare crisis may be to figure out how to keep everyone healthy [9, 10]?

The definition of *healthcare* by Merriam-Webster is: "efforts made to maintain or restore physical, mental, or emotional well-being especially by trained and licensed professionals." The first known use of the term was in 1940. We have become very adept at the *effort to restore* part, most likely because we are content to pay for something observable. In addition, there is universal acceptance of the expense to pay a health professional to do something for you, or to you. It is much harder to recognize the value of preventing an untoward event. How do we calculate or monitor the *effort to maintain*, and how do we pay for that. We know that at least 25% of the money attributed to "healthcare spending" has no effect on morbidity and mortality. But that is considered wasteful spending. It is difficult, if not impossible, to accurately determine the cost savings of good health. First, because we do not clearly understand what our current true "costs" are and, second, because if we eliminated preventable illness, would there be other illnesses to consider and pay for. Even under perfect conditions, perfect diet, appropriate prevention, and a lack of genetically acquired health conditions, the human body has a limited lifespan, due to physical and environmental stressors. Therefore, there will always be costs of treatment, even with the best prevention [11].

The term "reimburse," which is the common (but inappropriate) method of describing payment to a healthcare provider, has been intentionally omitted from this discussion of healthcare financing. Reimbursement suggests being repaid for something, such as being reimbursed for a business trip. This terminology has been applied to healthcare because it was considered unprofessional to discuss payment for services provided by a physician. No one speaks about reimbursing a plumber or an auto mechanic. We just pay the bill. However, there are myriads of articles written about physician reimbursement. If the discussion was honest, and the question posed was "How should we calculate physician payment," the problem becomes clear. We currently pay physicians to perform treatments and procedures – should we pay them instead to keep us healthy? Should everyone have equal access to care? YES. Should everyone have the ability to afford medications? YES. Should healthcare providers be appropriately compensated? YES. How can we afford this? **Keep people healthy!**

The following chapters develop concepts that are vital to a successful system of healthcare, one that focuses on health! I will try to avoid criticism of current practices without offering alternative solutions that are more aligned with the stated goal. However, it is impossible to propose change without critique of present inadequacies.

# 2

# Bending the Cost Curve

All of the changes in healthcare financing over the past 25 years (or longer) have had one goal in mind: bending the cost curve. Bending the curve implies lowering the annual increase in healthcare spending, not flattening the curve or decreasing annual spend. The prevailing perception is that there is a desire to decrease annual healthcare spending. This is erroneous and is perpetuated by an uninformed media. This is what drives the chatter about "death panels," rationing of care, and hospitals going bankrupt. Hospitals are supposed to serve their communities, and if a hospital closes, it is due to either poor management or a lack of need. This concept is similar to our public schools. They are built to serve the community and if they fail it is due to poor management or a lack of need. Schools are not part of our capitalist economic system and hospitals should not be either.

In every discussion comparing various other country's healthcare systems with ours, there is talk of outcomes, coverage, and access, but the major differentiator is cost. While most of the world has a relatively flat cost curve, the United States has a cost curve that continues to increase annually, even when looking at cost as a percentage of GDP (Gross Domestic Product). This is why the most important part of the Affordable Care Act (ACA) was capping the ceiling of healthcare spend to 14% of GDP. If spend increased over 14%, there was an automatic hold on all Federal healthcare spending, until GDP increased. Therefore, increased spending was allowed, as long as the rise was less than the rise in GDP. Even though the ACA has been eviscerated, there is still bipartisan support for "bending the curve" [12].

*Transforming Healthcare: An Insider's Look on Why and How*, First Edition. Morey Menacker.
© 2022 John Wiley & Sons, Inc. Published 2022 by John Wiley & Sons, Inc.
Companion website: www.wiley.com/go/menacker/transforminghealthcare

The introduction of Medicare Advantage was clearly part of the effort to bend the curve. Medicare Advantage is a system in which the Center for Medicare/Medicaid Services (CMS) provides an authorized private health plan with an annual stipend, as full payment, for providing comprehensive care to a Medicare patient who chooses this private option. The expectation is that there will be no need for the patient to require gap insurance nor a separate Part D policy. Federal regulations also allow these plans to offer other incentives to prospective patients, as long as they meet specific criteria set by CMS. This may include payment for certain over the counter items, limited or zero co-pay for PCP visits, transportation to medical visits, and other perks. These incentives must meet the scrutiny of CMS, but are used as selling points by the individual authorized health plans. The concept behind the program was to shift the financial risk to private insurers, along with the responsibility of case management and utilization management. CMS would monitor the plan to ensure that care was not restricted in any way, but CMS expenditures would be relatively fixed, based on a calculation of expected annual spend per patient, according to their reported severity of illness. While this would not necessarily change the total expenditure, it was felt that the private health plans would be better equipped to monitor spend via a utilization review. In 2016, there was discussion of eliminating Medicare Advantage, after the results were not seen as significantly bending the curve. There were other programs that seemed to have more success, and the penetration of Medicare Advantage plans in the Medicare aged population was limited. Most Medicare beneficiaries choose a traditional Medicare policy, and supplement with Part D, which assists in prescription costs. They may also choose to purchase "gap insurance," which covers the 20% of medical bills not covered under traditional Medicare policies [13].

Multiple provider organizations developed "models of care" in order to benefit financially from the Medicare Advantage (MA) program. Proposals for "shared risk" taking, encouraged those in Washington to continue the MA program. However, the ultimate goal for the government remained the same: Bend the Curve. The organizations that developed these new models recognized that there were two avenues available for financial success in MA: increased revenue and decreased expense. Revenue was dependent upon two factors, panel size and risk adjustment. Risk adjustment is the method in which CMS determines the predicted annual spend of an individual patient, and thereby the lump payment to the Health Plan. Panel size is determined by marketing. Decreasing the expense side is a much more difficult process. These organizations did not have a closed physician panel, and had to purchase certain services from hospitals, specialists, and health systems. There were a few exceptions, with organizations that maintained a closed system, owning all aspects of healthcare services: hospitals, physicians, outpatient diagnostics, pharmacy, and post-acute services. For those organizations that needed to "purchase" services, in addition to managing utilization, decreasing expenses also meant controlling patient behavior. For these reasons, the script developed by these provider organizations as a "model of care" suggested that working on the revenue side, or increasing CMS payment and increasing panel size, was the easiest and most logical path to financial success.

CMS adopted a method of Severity of Illness stratification, known as HCC, or Hierarchical Condition Category. This risk adjustment model is used to predict future healthcare costs and is used to augment the benchmark annual payment to the health plan managing the Medicare Advantage patient. CMS gathers the diagnoses from claims that are submitted by providers and hospitals. There are random audits performed by CMS to ensure that all diagnoses have corresponding support information. This is the intended obstacle to prevent risk-sharing provider organizations from gaming the system, or adding diagnoses in order to increase payment. As we have already discussed, the current payment model inappropriately (albeit innocently) rewards overutilization. This payment model rewards over diagnosis. If one wanted to maximize payment without regard for cost control, patient satisfaction, and outcome, tests would continually be ordered to increase the number of HCC diagnoses, without regard as to treatment and prevention of disease. In general, HCC diagnoses are limited to chronic problems that can affect mortality and morbidity. Acute problems are generally excluded, as the purpose is to calculate *future* expense. One must be vigilant to guarantee that the testing performed and the diagnoses added are purely to stratify health risk, and not to maximize payment. The terms *vigilant* and Federal Government are rarely found together in a sentence [14].

Another flaw in the HCC model is that many specialists add diagnoses to their billing in order to obtain authorizations for expensive, and sometimes unnecessary, testing. As mentioned before, in Medicare

Advantage, CMS gives full utilization management control to the health plan. Therefore, the health plan can decide if a procedure should be authorized for payment. Most specialists still function within the fee for service model, thereby benefiting from increased utilization. Authorization for a cardiac stress test may require a diagnosis of coronary artery disease, even though the test may be needed to diagnose the condition. However, providers are not allowed to use the term "rule out" in their billing. Therefore, the test will only be authorized, and paid, if a diagnosis of coronary artery disease exists. These diagnoses are forwarded to CMS and applied to the patient's HCC score. Actual examples of this process are too numerous to count, but can falsely change the HCC score for the patient, increasing payment, and cost to CMS.

There is faulty logic in the plan for risk-bearing organizations to focus solely on revenue, and ignore expense. Remember, the goal of the Medicare Advantage Program, and ALL federally sponsored healthcare initiatives, is to bend the cost curve. Increasing revenue may be a successful start for a small company, but to maintain success (and profit), one must be able to bend the curve. That means decreasing expense. While much more difficult to induce, the benefits are long lasting and reproducible. It also aids in the overarching goal of correcting our Healthcare Financing System, and secondarily fixing our Healthcare Delivery System. There is still benefit in accurately identifying Severity of Illness, and to maximize capitated distributions. However, the ultimate goal of any risk-sharing healthcare delivery organization MUST be bending the cost curve, utilizing primary, secondary, and tertiary prevention, coordinated with alignment of interests and patient education.

Over the past few years, Medicare Advantage has enrolled about 25% of all Medicare beneficiaries. This percentage is growing annually. Unfortunately, annually about 9% of MA patients disenroll from their current health plan. Most likely, the cause of these apparent unrelated statistics are probably one and the same; marketing from the Health Plans. The larger the patient panel, the more profit to the health plan. This is especially true if the provider organizations accept the downside financial risk. During the Annual Enrollment Period, the airwaves are inundated with advertisements from health plans, as well as health insurance brokers. These brokers get a commission for signing patients to a particular plan. Even if a patient is currently enrolled in Medicare Advantage, a broker receives a commission if they can convince the patient to change plans. These commissions are indirectly paid for by CMS, and are dollars that could be used (and should be used) for patient care. In addition to the monetary waste, a second problem associated with the high disenrollment rate is disjointed care. Oftentimes, when a patient changes plans, the broker will provide the patient with a different primary care doctor. This creates a situation where 9% of all Medicare Advantage patients see a new PCP annually, and have no continuity of care. It is also a disincentive for the health plans to focus on longitudinal prevention and care. They realize that it is not in their best interest to invest time and money in a patient who will move to another health plan in a year or two. There is no return on investment, as the next health plan will potentially see the decrease in expense generated by prevention. How is it acceptable that a government funded system rewards brokers for adversely affecting patient care? Clearly, the problem is the system, not the individuals [15].

Any future government action regarding healthcare financing will surely include provisions similar to the ACA, namely, tying spending to the GDP. Even in the unlikely event of a single payer system, the federal government must have a mechanism to control spending. If organizations can't profit from the management of Medicare patients, then increasing panel size only increases the loss. Any organization looking to the future must design a model that controls excessive healthcare spending. This includes controlling wasteful spending, the money spent that has no positive effect on patient outcome, morbidity, and mortality. It is estimated that over 25% of ALL healthcare spending can be considered wasteful. That does not mean that procedures are not performed, diagnostics are not done, medications are not prescribed. It means that all of these procedures, diagnostics, and medications do not help the patients. In addition to minimizing waste, it is imperative that we eliminate barriers to care, by taking responsibility for our patients, utilizing existing resources for those in need, and developing new programs to enhance access, make medication affordable, and educate our patients to take an active role in their health.

Spending on prevention is much more efficient than spending on treatment. The cost of preventing heart disease in an individual is much less than the cost for heart bypass surgery. However, patients are not accustomed to changing behavior if they feel well. A massive educational process must be developed to help patients understand the relationship between bad behavior and disease. This has been successful in the efforts to decrease cigarette use. In addition, providers are not currently trained to focus on prevention. While all the necessary knowledge is taught in medical school, the application of this knowledge is solely taught in the treatment of disease, or in the procedures used to diagnose disease. We cannot fault our doctors, as this has been driven by the method of financing healthcare. If you get paid to take care of sick people, you only treat sick people. It would be unusual for a butcher to recommend that you eat fish for dinner, or become a vegan.

The quickest way to bend the cost curve is to eliminate, or at least decrease, wasteful spending. This must be driven by eliminating the financial incentive of overutilization. In addition, every dollar of government funding must be accountable toward patient care, either directly or indirectly. Eventually, all the fat is cut away. By that time, we need to have developed a system of prevention, education, and support of social determinants, in order to decrease expenses related to preventable illness.

# 3

# Goals in Transforming Healthcare

What are the goals in the transformation of our healthcare system? The simplest answer is to look at the Quadruple Aim. For those uninitiated, the Quadruple Aim is the Triple Aim, plus one. The Triple Aim was first described by the Institute for Healthcare Improvement (IHI) in 2007. It included improving the patient experience, improving the health of our population as a whole, and reducing the per capita cost of healthcare. The Triple Aim was developed at the time it became obvious that our increase in per capita spending on healthcare was outpacing the GDP. The result was a consistent increase in the percentage of GDP attributed to healthcare, as well as an increase in the annual healthcare budget. Additionally, the general consensus by the public was that the US healthcare system was dysfunctional, substandard, and unaffordable. In order to ameliorate this untenable situation, the Triple Aim was accepted as a goal by CMS. This did not necessarily mean decreasing the total spending on healthcare; it meant a slowdown in the rapidly increasing rate of spending, while simultaneously improving the health of the population, as well as the patient experience [16, 17].

The IHI developed these concepts as a single plan, with simultaneous efforts at all three parameters. Patient experience not only addresses the issue of patient satisfaction, but also the need for the patient to be involved in decision-making, as well as have some accountability. Improving the health of populations not only requires quality medical care, but includes minimizing, or eliminating, the barriers to healthy living – the so-called Social Determinants. This also must include identifying and mitigating environmental factors for disease and holding the population accountable for habits that lead to increased morbidity

*Transforming Healthcare: An Insider's Look on Why and How*, First Edition. Morey Menacker.
© 2022 John Wiley & Sons, Inc. Published 2022 by John Wiley & Sons, Inc.
Companion website: www.wiley.com/go/menacker/transforminghealthcare

and mortality. Decreasing per capita spending would be a natural result of improved health of our population, but also must take into account the enormous amount of money spent in healthcare that have no positive effect on health, also termed wasteful spending. Unfortunately, our physician training programs focus on treatment of disease, not prevention. This is due primarily to two seemingly unrelated, yet intertwined, causes. First, the field of Preventive Medicine is only a recently recognized specialty and, for most medical schools, a single course discussing vaccinations and screening tests. Second, our payment system has developed to compensate for treatment, and the more invasive and complex the treatment, the greater the payment. This system of payment is a direct descendent of the establishment of Medicare. While physicians have embraced the system, and participated in "reform" of the payment system, it is a government system that was the driving force. It therefore seems rational to propose that Preventive Medicine was only recently recognized because there was no payment for it.

The Quadruple Aim maintains the three tenets of the Triple Aim, but included healthcare workforce satisfaction. It has become clear that providers, staff, and care teams must feel happy for healthcare organizations to achieve and sustain improved patient outcomes. The effort required in achieving the Triple Aim requires total commitment by government, health plans, patients, and healthcare workers. In order to prevent burnout, many in the healthcare community replaced the Triple Aim with the Quadruple Aim [16, 17].

The Quadruple Aim is not four independent goals; there is significant overlap as these goals are interdependent. For example, if the goal of cost control was addressed without concern for patient outcome or patient satisfaction, treatments could be denied that would have an effect on outcome. On the other hand, if we allow patients to request diagnostics and treatments that may not be appropriate, or worse, contraindicated, for the purpose of their "satisfaction," then cost and outcomes are adversely affected. Another way of looking at the goal of transforming healthcare is to make sure that the patient receives the right care, at the right location, at the right time, by the right provider. Unfortunately, this does not take into account the responsibility of the patient as an active participant in preventing illness and controlling chronic disease. While this is a noble goal for providers of healthcare, it ignores the patient's place in this process.

What do we mean by mandating the "right care, in the right place, by the right person"? It has been reported that medical errors account for 10% of all deaths in the United States, the third leading cause behind heart disease and cancer. These can be errors of commission, such as the wrong medicine being prescribed or dispensed, the wrong dosage, surgical errors, misdiagnoses, etc. There are also errors of omission, such as the inability to pick up warning signs from a patient's history, a lack of knowledge by the provider, leading to a delay in appropriate treatment, or the use of antiquated treatment regimens due to inadequate continuing education. In this era of provider compensation driven by volume, there is little time to research current trends, to ponder a diagnosis or treatment plan, or to immerse oneself in the current state of medical knowledge. We depend upon our providers to be knowledgeable in the diseases they are treating, but where is the oversight, the mandate to "do no harm?" With computers everywhere and instant ability to research even the most arcane topics, why are providers not using these tools to minimize mistakes in diagnosis and treatment? Why is this information not readily accessible, updated regularly, and mandatory to utilize? Taking this concept a step further, why don't we have readily accessible outcomes data for providers, hospitals, healthcare organizations, and treatments? If a patient were diagnosed with Prostate Cancer, shouldn't he have the right, based upon data, to determine what treatment is best, such as surgery, external beam radiation, internal radiation seeds, proton therapy, hormonal therapy, or no treatment? Currently, the decision is driven by a provider who may or may not have a financial motivation to choose one treatment over another. And once the treatment is chosen, shouldn't the patient have the information available to choose the best individual to provide this treatment? Additionally, doesn't every patient deserve to receive the most appropriate treatment for their illness? It is impossible for any provider to have the entirety of the world's knowledge of medicine memorized, but today's technology and computing power can provide this. Why isn't it commonplace [18]?

When designing a new system of healthcare, we cannot create a system only for those who can afford it, or those who are working, or any other attempt at limiting access to care. The transformation of our healthcare system must provide access for everyone. This includes access to providers, access to medications, and access to appropriate diagnostics and therapeutics. As social determinants play a large role in the incidence and the progression of disease, access to appropriate food, clothing, and shelter must also be provided. It must be emphasized that in order to participate in this system, there are patient responsibilities to be acknowledged. Behaviors that are counterproductive to health must be addressed. Behavioral health issues must be addressed. Patient education is a mandatory accessory to all healthcare interactions. Patients must know what to do, as well as why, how, when, and where.

Our current system of healthcare promotes a transactional relationship between patient and provider. In general, patients see providers in order to receive treatment, receive medical advice, or receive recommendations for diagnostics, therapeutics, or specialty services. In return, the provider receives payment, usually from a third party. There is no trust built, no ownership of the issue/problem, and no responsibility, or interest, in the outcome. In an uncomfortable way, our current system promotes providers to keep patients ill, and does not promote prevention or patient accountability. This was never the intended outcome, but merely an unintended consequence of the financial system built to support the healthcare industry. Alternatively, the goal of the transformed healthcare system must be development of a trusting relationship between patient and provider, as well as shared responsibility for prevention of disease, amelioration of symptoms, and control of chronic illness. In this manner, dollars currently utilized to treat preventable conditions, or to pay for unnecessary testing and interventions, could be shifted to provide care to those currently unable to afford "personalized care," and therefore over-utilize emergency services and hospitals. However, those treatments come with an added, unrecognized cost – the expense of emergency and hospital services performed on uninsured (or underinsured) individuals are cost shifted to those with insurance, thereby increasing the average cost of care for everyone.

It is imperative that in order to understand the financial aspects of transforming healthcare, we recognize the amount of emergency and hospital services that could have been prevented with primary care intervention, early recognition of disease, patient education, and access to care. Every hospital maintains an emergency plan to initiate should there be a natural disaster in their community. Under this plan, the clinicians at the hospital evaluate all current patients, and determine which patients could be sent home, or to a lower level of care, such as a subacute nursing facility. If there are patients who could be treated equally well at home or at a lower cost facility, then why are they currently in the hospital? The answer is similar to the response given by John Dillinger when asked why he robbed banks – "because that's where the money is."

The goals for the transformation of healthcare must include the quadruple aim, a focus on prevention of illness, and active participation in health maintenance by patients; all driving a bend in the healthcare cost curve. The value of something is defined by its worth, what we are willing to spend for it, either in money, in effort, or in time. If something is free it has minimal or no value, but freedom itself has an incalculable value. Free healthcare has no inherent value, but being healthy for life has an incalculable value.

# 4

# Quality, Efficiency, Outcomes, and Access

Defining quality is very similar to defining pornography; "I can't explain it, but I know it when I see it!" As an intern, I was performing a History and Physical examination on a patient in the hospital. I saw that her Primary Care Physician (PCP) was a provider who was "known" at the hospital as providing poor quality care. When I asked her why she chose him as her PCP, she answered quickly, "He must be good because his office is always crowded and he charges more than all the other doctors in town." I later learned that this provider had family members sit in his waiting room early in his practice, to appear busier than he was.

Quality medical care may sometimes involve a surgical intervention, a change in medication, a diagnostic test, a referral to a specialist, instructive patient education, or even watchful waiting. Conversely, each of the above choices could be listed as poor medical care, depending upon the situation. Quality may be viewed as providing the "right" care to the patient, but sometimes, with additional information, that choice may turn out to be the "wrong" care. For example, a patient who presents with a Strep throat would best be treated with a course of a penicillin antibiotic. However, what if the patient has a history of severe allergy to penicillin? While this seems to be an unlikely experience, as most of us know if we are intolerant to penicillin, there are a myriad of treatments that can be damaging to patients with specific medical histories, which may go unnoticed. Therefore, quality must also include an appropriate exploration of all data that can affect the medical decision-making. The term "appropriate" is key because, occasionally, an exhaustive battery of tests can delay treatment, and also dramatically increase the cost of care.

*Transforming Healthcare: An Insider's Look on Why and How*, First Edition. Morey Menacker.
© 2022 John Wiley & Sons, Inc. Published 2022 by John Wiley & Sons, Inc.
Companion website: www.wiley.com/go/menacker/transforminghealthcare

If we define quality as the "right" choice after a comprehensive review, are we any closer to an answer? This does not take into account decisions that are made under emergency circumstances. At times, decisions are made by providers with limited information, due to the critical status of the patient and the need to provide treatment immediately. Therefore, we need to make the "right" decision, after comprehensive review, if possible, but with speed and accuracy when needed. This process requires an ability to rapidly assess a situation, gather whatever information is available, and create a plan of intervention based upon an accurate risk–benefit calculation. An example of this process in action is the response to an event in an Emergency Department, either due to trauma or a catastrophic event such as cardiac arrest or shock.

When evaluating the quality of medical care, one can utilize "best practice" standards as an appropriate bar to achieve. All physician organizations, from primary care to specialties, produce annual guidelines of care for a multitude of diseases. These guidelines are constantly reviewed and updated, based upon new data from research, new treatments available, and new diagnostics. As a group, they are referred to as Practice Guidelines, or Best Practice Guidelines. Quality medical care requires adherence to the practice guidelines for the disease being treated. The treatment of congestive heart failure is different in 2020 than it was in 2010 or 2000. It is the responsibility of providers to remain current in the treatment of all diseases that they manage, yet there is little or no oversight that this occurs. While it is true that all licensed providers are required to partake in continuing medical education, much of this is performed for the purpose of maintaining licensure, as opposed to improved decision making, updating the knowledge base, and ensuring quality. Additionally, most, if not all, medical specialties require a recertification examination. However, there are many intensive courses available for a physician to prepare and pass the examination, similar to a high school student preparing for a college entrance examination. The new information is used to pass an examination, and does not necessarily change practice patterns. More consideration must be taken in the evaluation of physician quality, both in the hospital and in the office setting. In a provider's office, there is no requirement to provide the most up to date treatment, or even to limit practice to specific areas of expertise. Physicians are licensed to practice "Medicine and Surgery", and in their private office there is no training requirement. As outrageous as it may seem, a medical provider may perform whatever procedure, or treat whatever disease process, which they feel comfortable with. Unless a complaint is forwarded to the state's Board of Medical Examiners, there is no oversight. Most often, any adverse outcomes are identified through patient reporting, or litigation. Within a hospital setting, there are committees to review quality, but rarely are there serious discussions about the standard of care unless an adverse event occurs. Health plans only seem to get involved when a request is made for an expensive test or treatment. Quality appears to be measured by health plans solely as an extension of cost.

The relationship between cost and quality is complicated. While many consumers feel that the cost of a product correlates directly with the product's quality, this is not always the case. In fact, when discussing the cost of healthcare, more often than not there is a poor correlation between quality and cost. At this time, it is appropriate to digress into a discussion of cost within the healthcare world.

It is nearly impossible to ascertain the true cost of healthcare. This is because healthcare accounting does not function as a cost-based system. The system is based on "charges" allowed by CMS and all commercial health insurers calculate allowable fees charged as a percentage of Medicare. CMS has set fees for all possible codes, both Evaluation and Management codes and Procedure codes. All private health insurance companies negotiate rate schedules with doctors and hospitals based on a percent of the Medicare fee schedule. In general, the fee schedule of private health plans is higher than that of Medicare. These increased fees are then used to offset the lack of payment by those patients without health insurance coverage. Commercial insurers have little concern for true cost, because any unexpected expense is automatically added to the calculation of the next year's premium. Hospital organizations only look at global expenses versus total revenue generated by billing. There are significant expenses associated with maintaining a functioning hospital, and the costs associated are not analyzed with respect of the specific payment for the services performed. If an individual walked into a hospital and asked the cost of an MRI, because he wanted to pay cash, he could be told the charge, but not the actual cost. This situation exists with every possible hospitalization, surgery, diagnostic test, etc. Most organizations have no idea of their cost per procedure, including all direct and indirect costs. Conversely, almost all hotels know exactly the cost of each room per night, all airlines know the cost of each seat in the plane, and so forth. In reality, when the first MRI (magnetic resonance imaging) machine was opened for clinical use, the charge attached was an arbitrary number. This number has never been adjusted downward, in relation to increased volume. The added revenue generated by that increasing volume becomes profit. This is why hospitals compete for the highest paying procedures, such as heart surgery, transplant, oncology treatment, etc. They do not know if there is profit in a specific procedure, just that the payment is high. They also do not know for certain if the direct and indirect expense associated with that procedure makes it profitable or a loss leader.

Returning to the discussion of cost as a factor of quality, we must look at the issue of medical devices. If a patient requires a total hip replacement, what is the criteria for selecting which company's product is used? The answer almost always is that the surgeon chooses what medical device company should be used and the hospital purchases the prosthesis, in order to keep the surgeon's "business." How does the surgeon choose the company? That is much more complicated. While it is illegal to receive money for choosing one company over another, it is commonplace for these companies to "employ" doctors as speakers, advisors, and representatives. This can be very rewarding for all parties, except those of us stuck with the bill. This same process occurs with cardiac devices, medical equipment, surgical implants, and even cataract lenses. The most costly choice is not necessarily the highest quality product. Cost also should not be the only criteria used by hospital purchasing. However, the specter of individual monetary gain must not be utilized in these decisions.

This process of physician participation is commonly reproduced within the pharmaceutical industry. In addition, pharmaceutical companies spend hundreds of millions advertising directly to the consumer. There are a myriad of commercials for rheumatoid arthritis treatments every evening during prime-time viewing. There seem to be more advertisements than patients requiring treatment. Imagine the profit margin in the sale of these medications, if the cost of the commercials is considered a mere overhead. Has anyone asked the actual cost to produce the treatment? The pharmaceutical industry has created an entire advertising sector, generating revenue under the guise of "healthcare costs." Who could have known that advertising agencies, and actors' salaries, could be considered healthcare expenses? These costs to the pharmaceutical industry have been built into the price of the medications, which are clearly included when calculating healthcare costs.

It is apparent that if the plan is to move the financial risk of quality medical care to the healthcare provider (or organization), then the issue of excessive cost for secondary gain by providers becomes a moot point. The fees generated by these providers would be automatically added to their expense line, negating the financial gain. However, a model that rewards ancillary businesses based on the quality of their products, and limits exorbitant markups, is required to control wasteful spending, in a system fraught with such waste.

The issue of quality, and adherence to standards, is a bit murkier. If an organization focuses entirely on expenses, then how do we ensure that quality is not lost in the quest for the bottom line? Clearly, improved outcomes would be a good measure of quality. However, in some situations, outcomes cannot be measured immediately. For example, the complications associated with diabetes can take fifteen years to appear. In order to determine quality diabetic care by evaluating the outcomes would become a lifetime task. Another measurement of quality must be considered. This conundrum actually provides an opportunity.

It is currently standard practice for all healthcare providers to utilize electronic medical records. This process was accelerated with federal subsidies for electronic medical record (EMR) adoption. Unfortunately, there was no concurrent mandate that these programs have interoperability, or be able to speak to one another. The federal government, in their haste to move the healthcare establishment into the computer age, actually created a veritable Tower of Babel for healthcare. Many of the so-called EMRs were no more than glorified word processing programs. Most information shared between providers were stored as PDFs, or pictures, and were not actionable items, minimizing any data analysis provided by the EMR. Without the ability to analyze data, these electronic records were merely typed notes that were being stored in a file cabinet. The inherent value of electronic medical records is to analyze trends, optimize treatment, and minimize errors, both of omission and commission. This value is minimized by the use of health records that are essentially snapshots placed in an album.

It is important to understand that not only are the best practice standards available to be integrated with any EMR, but, if comprehensive data are available, can direct the provider in real time as to the proper diagnostic direction, or treatment modality. To be blunt, if our EMRs could share data, and we utilized best practice guidelines, our computers would have the capability of recommending the best course of action, and even prohibit decisions that could have adverse effects. A major part of healthcare transformation MUST include not only the ability to provide quality care but also a monitoring system to ensure quality care. Our current technology has this capability; we just need the desire/ responsibility/intention/drive/reason to utilize, and to mandate it.

Another aspect of quality involves personalization. Every year, there is more information as to how our genetic makeup affects disease acquisition, disease severity, and disease treatment. The more information we have about a patient, the better we can personalize diagnostic and treatment recommendations. As providers gripe about how treatment guidelines correspond to "cookbook medicine," the necessity to identify and document specific individual idiosyncrasies raises the bar on the responsibility and skill of the provider. An entire branch of research, called Precision Medicine, is exploding and will help drive the future of healthcare. Precision medicine is a recognition that individuals respond differently to various stressors, as well as treatments. Much of this is related to our specific genetic makeup, but much also may be related to our anatomy, our physiology, our age, our environment, and our concurrent conditions. It is common for pediatric patients to receive a smaller dose of medicine than an adult would require, but this is entirely due to the medication and the disease being treated. Occasionally, children require a higher dosage to achieve the desired results. We are learning that certain genes can alter the efficacy of some medications, as well as the decision as to which medication to use. This is becoming a common event in the treatment of cancer and it is likely that it will become more common in all disease treatment. Under our current payment model, the driver for personalized service is increased charges; in the proposed model, the driver will be improved quality and outcome.

Efficiency is an interesting concept when it is related to healthcare. Efficiency can be boiled down to receiving the right care, at the right location, at the right time, by the right provider. While many would condemn the Canadian Health System as inefficient because of potential delays in elective surgery, those delays may make them more efficient in caring for patients with urgent problems. For example, a patient in Canada requiring hip replacement may have to wait weeks to months for the surgery to be scheduled. In the United States, this surgery is scheduled as soon as possible, but for what reason? Could it be because the surgeon and the hospital are paid handsomely for the procedure? Efficiency should be evaluated on the basis of timing of care. If a treatment is required urgently, is this accomplished? Were unnecessary tests performed? Was the "cost" appropriate for the outcome? This definition of cost includes the monetary aspect, the effect on the hip surgery patient for preventing delay in treatment and recovery, and the effect on the healthcare system for prioritizing high paying procedures. We must try to quantify the benefit to the patient for receiving rapid treatment, beyond the patient satisfaction criteria. Was the patient benefitted by pain relief, improved mobility, independent ADLs (activities of daily living), and, if so, what is that worth in dollars? Did the healthcare system shift resources in order to accommodate this procedure? Could these resources have been used elsewhere to positively affect other patients? Was an urgent surgery delayed in order to allow this high paying elective procedure to be performed expeditiously? The current US financing system does not align with this model of efficiency, and clearly is not aligned with positive outcomes.

Another aspect of efficiency that goes unnoticed is the propensity to order diagnostic tests. While the value of certain diagnostic tests cannot be questioned, a common occurrence seems to be that "what's wrong with the test is what's wrong with the patient." This is magnified in the Emergency Departments of many hospitals. The volume of patients has driven many providers of emergency care to order tests based on patient complaints, and not based upon focused history taking and physical examination. Many hospital radiologists have shared that their reports should read, "Normal findings, cleared for History and Physical." Diagnostic testing should be used to confirm or rule out a specific condition or disease under consideration, following comprehensive evaluation. However, since diagnostic tests are handsomely compensated, many providers feel that it is appropriate to perform an abundance of tests, rationalizing that "no one is paying for it" or "the information is beneficial." Routine testing has never been shown to alter mortality, morbidity, or outcome. The benefits are purely monetary, and, with changes to the financing system, will become extinct.

When reviewing treatment options for any patient, it would seem obvious that cost, efficiency, and positive outcomes would be prominent in decision making. However. we pay for the "service" and unconsciously expect the system to provide cost, efficiency, and outcome measures. As noted above, we are lacking in our intention to quantify cost and efficiency. It seems rather simple to quantify positive outcomes. If the patient improves, then the outcome is positive. However, what is the incentive for focus on positive outcomes? Not only is our current payment system agnostic to outcome, on occasion a positive outcome is a disincentive. Hospitals are paid to keep their beds full; an empty bed is an expense to them. Emergency rooms and trauma services are significant expenses to hospitals. If they are not utilized, the expense remains, but there is no revenue to offset the cost. Another example is the patient who presents to the dermatologist with a skin cancer. The doctor may perform an excision of the cancer in the office and close the wound. However, there is a procedure known as MOHS (devised by C.H. Mohs), in which the cancer is removed in thin slices, with each slice being examined under the microscope for evidence of cancer cells. Once complete, the patient then requires a second surgery to close the defect caused by the procedure. While this process is indicated in facial cancers, to limit the amount of tissue removed and minimize disfigurement, the procedure is charged at a rate of 10–50 times that of the minor excision. Dermatologists routinely recommend this procedure for ALL skin cancers, and not because of better outcomes.

A final point about positive outcomes is that, many times, outcomes can take years to become apparent. One of the most common chronic illnesses is diabetes. As previously noted, complications associated with diabetes, such as kidney disease, heart disease, vascular and neurologic disease, can take 15–20 years to develop. The average length of time, currently, that an individual remains with a specific health plan is 16 months. If the health plan knows that their coverage will be limited in time, why should they focus on a prevention plan that they, the insurer, will not benefit from? Why should a hospital system spend money (profits) today in order to prevent illness 15–20 years from now? C-suiters only care about this year's profit/loss statement. There is no sound financial reason, in the current healthcare finance model, to spend money on prevention. That is why the current system of healthcare financing must change.

Not only must outcome measurement be an integral part of oversight in the transformed healthcare system, but a method to ensure continuity of care must be included. As mentioned above, healthcare insurers only expect the average patient (they call them beneficiaries) to remain in their control for 16 months. This occurs because most health insurers are for-profit companies and must answer to their shareholders. If their profit per beneficiary is limited to 15%, as in Obamacare, the only avenue to increase profit is to increase market share. Therefore, the companies promote new business by offering lower premiums for the first year (in the commercial market) or increased covered services (in the Medicare Advantage market). That allows the companies to predict growth in covered lives every year and elevates the stock price. We do not see the same process in the life insurance market. People tend to purchase life insurance and stay with the same company for many years. This is because there are financial incentives for a person to maintain the same life insurance. Why can't the same model be utilized in the health insurance market?

Why is it important for patients to have the same insurance provider? This allows the patient to remain with the same healthcare organization that is taking the financial risk for the care of the patient. Continuity of care decreases cost, decreases unnecessary testing, improves efficiency, and helps to drive preventive measures. If a healthcare organization knows they will be financially responsible for a patient's care for many years, every effort to prevent or minimize disease will be undertaken early and often, in order to ensure financial stability. Clearly, patients must maintain the ability to choose their healthcare provider, but it must be made with full knowledge of the provider's quality, efficiency, and outcome data. Choosing a provider based on advertising, incentives, or coercion is unacceptable. Coercion can occur when an insurance broker benefits from recommending a specific provider in the market. This is not relevant in a single payer system, however, as the financial strength of the health insurance industry suggests that a single payer system is not part of our future reality [19, 20].

Access to care is an inherent responsibility of any healthcare system. If care is not accessible, then quality, efficiency, and outcomes suffer. As hospitals and emergency rooms are always open and functioning, the only issue with access to these facilities is cost, which has already been discussed. However, in our transformed system, prevention is a major focus regarding cost control. This prevention requires interaction and education by primary care providers. Most primary care providers maintain office hour availability during regular working hours, Monday through Friday. For patients who work full time, this schedule discourages preventive visits, as it would require days off from work. This creates dissatisfaction. It appears that providers create their work schedules for their own benefit, and not the benefit of the client (patient). Routine outpatient specialty services can also be inconvenient for patients. It is vital in a transformed system to provide services directed at the convenience of the patient population, in order to maximize utilization and ensure success.

Another aspect in the realm of access is the high cost of pharmaceuticals. It seems ludicrous that a patient can be diagnosed with a condition, yet not be able to afford the proper treatment. How can the pharmaceutical industry be immune from governmental regulation, especially when people's lives are at risk? In fact, how can we condone inaccessibility of a treatment, due to excessive cost, when the resulting negative outcome will command much higher costs, in hospitalization, health, and wellbeing? It seems clear that any transformation of the healthcare system must include the pharmaceutical industry, encouraging innovation while containing cost. Entrepreneurship can be encouraged, but not at the expense of provision of services.

**5**

# Overcoming Inertia

Any discussion regarding transforming healthcare requires a conversation about overcoming inertia. "Why," you may ask, "do we need to discuss physics?" Inertia is defined as *a tendency to do nothing*, which may be an apropos term for a myriad of societal problems. However, in physics, inertia is defined as *a property of matter by which it continues in its existing state of rest, unless that state is changed by an external force.* By adding the caveat, that to overcome inertia, an external force is required, clarifies the difficulty in attempting change, under any circumstances. When we are dealing with issues that involve governmental action, the term "difficulty" yields to improbability, and even impossibility. It is true that the natural history of any and all things document slow, subtle, change that is relatively constant, and oblivious to most observers. This type of slow movement can be measured in years, generations, epochs, centuries, or millennia. Acceptance of the belief that our healthcare system is fundamentally flawed, and requires significant alteration, does not warrant glacial change, but dramatically different thinking. Glacial change is unacceptable in our current healthcare environment. The change needed will require an external force comprised of will, energy, education, diversity, and fortitude. There are many powerful organizations that do not want any substantial change to our healthcare system. Not that they are fearful of change, but they have become successful by developing systems that have generated huge profits in the name of medical treatment, and are not interested, and unwilling, to alter their business models [21].

*Transforming Healthcare: An Insider's Look on Why and How*, First Edition. Morey Menacker.
© 2022 John Wiley & Sons, Inc. Published 2022 by John Wiley & Sons, Inc.
Companion website: www.wiley.com/go/menacker/transforminghealthcare

This is not a critique of successful business practices. It merely is a statement of fact that many companies have become successful by modeling their business plans to maximize profit in the name of health. While our capitalist economy rewards entrepreneurship and profit, it has come at the expense of access to care, financial stability, and the health of our population as a whole. If a private for-profit company took over the policing of our country, and generated huge profits for its investors, would we be aghast? Of course we would. If private industry took over public education in our country, increasing cost and generating huge profit, would we be tolerant? Of course not. But this is the current state of our healthcare system. We have for-profit hospitals and nursing facilities, pharmaceutical companies, and medical device makers generating ungodly profits, clinical laboratories bribing physicians to use their labs due to the outrageous markups, and financial and tech giants announcing that they are planning to "disrupt" the healthcare industry. "Disrupt" is code for stealing some of the profits.

It is obvious that these organizations do not want to change our current healthcare system. However, this list is merely the tip of an iceberg, and the goal of transforming healthcare is the equivalent of the Titanic.

One organization resistant to change is the medical community, the providers of healthcare services. A common argument by physicians against change is that they prefer independence and do not wish to become hourly employees or practice "cookbook" medicine. Cookbook medicine is a derogatory term coined by physicians who feel that they do not want to be told what treatment is best for a certain condition. The argument is that the practice of medicine is an art, blended with science. In our current payment system, almost all physicians receive their compensation from an insurance provider, either private or governmental. Therefore, the independence argument holds no water. Almost all providers of healthcare services are paid via some third party. In addition, compensation for most services is predetermined by payment schedules. The providers may have the independence to decide where they practice, but are beholden to others for their compensation. In regards to "cookbook" medicine, it is an established fact that patient outcomes are optimized when providers utilize standards of care, developed by research and experts in the field. The argument therefore seems to be that physicians either do not want to provide the best care for their patients, or they are fearful that they currently are not providing the best possible care. Neither answer is acceptable nor valid. However, in actuality, the medical community carries little force and its inertia can be easily overcome.

The health insurance industry has significant risk with any drastic changes to our healthcare finance system. If the country moved to a single payer, nationalized healthcare financing system, the insurance industry would no longer exist in its current state. If the multipayer model was maintained, there would need to be limits placed on profit, marketing, and utilization of services. The plans would sign members and then transfer the premiums to organizations who would manage care and take financial risk. Some of these companies may decide to become provider organizations themselves. This would be a difficult transition to accomplish successfully. Our current model of health insurance develops premium pricing based upon risk stratification and actuarial tables, similar to life insurance. The companies then focus on volume as the driver of profit. A conversion to a care delivery organization would require a dramatic shift in philosophy, as success is determined by outcomes and efficiency, two words currently not available in any insurance vocabulary.

The major forces in our health insurance industry are publicly traded, for-profit companies, which depend upon future growth to drive the stock price. If the profit margin is fixed, and excess dollars are used to fill social gaps, these behemoths would essentially become public utilities. It is a fine business, with guaranteed returns, but is not acceptable for companies that have operating revenues greater than most countries. The insurance industry funded the public relations campaign that doomed the Clinton healthcare plan and almost derailed Obamacare. It seems reasonable to think that these companies will mount a serious attack on any change in our healthcare financing system, thereby increasing inertia.

The medical device industry enjoys enormous freedom in the current environment. They have the ability to create price structures that are paid by hospitals and healthcare organizations, and then billed to the insurers. These "costs" are then passed on to the consumer in the form of higher premiums or co-pays. Why wouldn't an organization shop for the most reasonably priced device? Because the manufacturers have created a model where the physician demands a specific device to be available, in order to bring his patient to their hospital for the procedure. Since the hospitals focus on the high DRG procedures, they purchase what the physician requests, in order to boost volume. Since the hospitals don't absorb the price of the device, but pass it along, their investment is minimal. Why would a physician demand a specific brand? There are a multitude of reasons, including the fact that many device makers provide training to physicians on the performance of highly compensated procedures. In addition, many physicians become "expert speakers" for the manufacturers, as well as highly paid trainers of new recruits. Much of this "wasteful spending" will disappear under the recommended payment reform, which focuses on health and prevention. Since the cost of medical devices will be borne by the care delivery organization, such organizations will shop for the highest quality at the lowest price. Physicians will be compensated for the care they provide, not per procedure. It is clear that physician compensation must be incentivized to drive the highest quality care, not the highest cost care. In addition, prevention will be compensated as high as intervention, thereby changing the focus to prevention of disease, from treatment of disease. The medical device industry will continue to be profitable as the need for new technology will not wane. However, cost control of these medical devices should provide significant savings to the healthcare system as a whole. It is clear that the medical device industry would prefer the status quo, adding to inertia against change.

The pharmaceutical industry has been viewed as the "evil empire" by many who espouse healthcare reform. It is true that pharma generates huge profits while utilizing patents to control the market. On the other hand, the pharmaceutical industry has provided enormous advances in the treatment of disease, and their ongoing research is vital to improving the health of our society. However, it is inappropriate for the United States to shoulder the entire cost of research and development, while the rest of the world purchases the same medications at much lower prices, either due to contracts or price controls. This problem cannot be solved without some level of governmental oversight. In addition, much of the direct advertising to the consumer must be reined in, with the average American believing that the advertised medication will change their life, and demand it by name! In the future, one would expect (and demand) that every patient will receive the best treatment for their problems, without the need for mass marketing.

The emerging development of immunologic agents being successful in the treatment of many diseases, most notably cancer and rheumatologic disorders, has dramatically altered the landscape of the pharmaceutical industry. These medications have been priced at astronomical levels, but their efficacy in treating previously chronic or terminal conditions has driven utilization despite the costs. These prices have had a dramatic impact upon health insurance, hospitals, as well as patients. While it is understandable that the cost of research must be recouped, the prices of these treatments has driven some patients into bankruptcy, and has caused insurance companies to attempt to withhold lifesaving treatment based upon cost. The only winners appear to be the stockholders, and the lawyers, who take pleasure in litigation. Either way, the patient winds up the loser. We must create a fair pricing model that allows and encourages innovation, while preventing care from being limited to only those with the financial means.

This discussion will not be complete without a comment regarding the greatest obstruction to change – our elected representatives in Washington. Our society has created a model in which elected officials have only one priority: to remain in power. Rhetoric aside, from the day they take office, our representatives begin campaigning to remain in office. This includes fundraising, political action committees, and avoiding controversy. The enormous amount of influence carried by the health insurance industry and the pharmaceutical industry is directly related to the amount of money spent by them on lobbying and political action. This influence is magnified by the public relations efforts aimed at maintaining the status quo. Until our elected representatives are shielded from influencers, inertia will prevent transformation. Additionally, it has become clear that our friends in Washington are more interested in the "sound bite" than in driving change. Every discussion regarding healthcare is utilized by our elected representatives as an opportunity to assure their constituents that they will defend the Constitution and protect us all from harm. If any idea is raised by a member of the opposition party, it must be bad for the country! This rancor can be termed an "inertia multiplier."

The final obstacle to overcoming inertia is the American public. Most people are very comfortable with the healthcare they currently receive, and are blind to the suffering of others. Fear of losing what they already have is a great motivator against change. The public has learned not to trust the government, not to trust politicians, and not to trust that someone else cares about them. They don't want to give up the "bird in hand" for the "two in the bush." As there is a financial element to all change, most people are risk averse, and would rather let things stay the same. Seniors do not want to give up their Medicare benefits, employees don't want to give up their employer sponsored health insurance, and those uninsured have little if no voice.

It is an utmost priority to educate the public about the inefficiencies of our current system, and the lack of attention to health. This new model of care must be marketed in a similar fashion as the latest perfume, cars, clothing, and other consumer products. The public must demand that healthcare focus on the health of the population, not the illnesses that pay the highest commission. People must understand that we can have it both ways: the best system of treating disease (when necessary) AND the best system to prevent illness and suffering. We currently enjoy the first, but are severely lagging the rest of the civilized world in the second.

# 6

## Patient Accountability

Our current fee for service model of care promotes the concept of the patient as a passive observer, moving from doctor to doctor, hospital to skilled nursing facility, without any role in decision-making nor responsibility for their own behavior, which may have been a factor in their disease or illness. The common perception of the public is that medical providers are available to take care of you when you are sick. Some people will go to see a medical provider for monitoring a chronic condition, but the number of patients who see providers for preventive care is minute. There are multiple rationales for this behavior. Many people do not want to "look for trouble" and are apprehensive about preventive screening. Many are afraid of the medical profession and avoid physicians at all costs. Many are concerned about the high cost of healthcare and either have a high deductible health plan or a plan that does not cover preventive testing.

With the patient as a passive observer to their care, the responsibility for maintaining health, or a return to health, is solely in the hands of the provider of services. The concept of the patient as a passive observer allows providers to order tests, perform procedures, prescribe medications and treatments, and even perform surgery, without concern for appropriateness, quality, or cost. In general, "someone else is paying for it," so why worry? The more tests performed, the greater the compensation. Preventive care and patient education do not pay well, so it is not prioritized by physicians. In addition, physicians are not trained in preventive care; they are trained to diagnose and treat disease. Part of the blame for overutilization of diagnostic testing, overutilization of hospital inpatient services, and overutilization of surgical services belongs to the

*Transforming Healthcare: An Insider's Look on Why and How*, First Edition. Morey Menacker.
© 2022 John Wiley & Sons, Inc. Published 2022 by John Wiley & Sons, Inc.
Companion website: www.wiley.com/go/menacker/transforminghealthcare

providers. However, there is a component of responsibility that lies at the feet of the patient. In reality, WE ARE ALL PAYING FOR THIS, either directly or indirectly through insurance premiums, taxes, and increased cost of goods and services, to cover employer-sponsored health insurance expenses or to pay for the services of uninsured patients.

Additionally, certain human behaviors put one at increased risk for health problems. Obvious issues like cigarette smoking, substance abuse, alcohol abuse, and obesity carry significant risks. However, failure to appropriately vaccinate, failure to perform primary, secondary, or tertiary prevention, and failure to adhere to provider recommendations also carry certain risks. Primary prevention includes avoidance of health hazards, either individually or as a society, and prevention due to immunizations. Examples would include smoking avoidance, healthy eating, and exercising, or more complex issues such as regulation and elimination of dangerous chemicals, seat belt laws, and child car seats. While many would argue that they have the right to behave as they see fit, public health laws prevent individuals from behaviors that could adversely affect another's wellbeing. This is the rationale behind smoking bans, automobile inspections, child seatbelt laws, etc. In fact, we currently have laws preventing people with known communicable diseases from public spaces. Patients with tuberculosis who are refusing treatment can be quarantined at home, or even imprisoned, until they complete treatment, and are no longer a risk to others. While this aggressive action is not condoned for those refusing primary prevention, shouldn't everyone bear some obligation to try to be healthy and limit healthcare expenses [22]?

Secondary prevention consists of screening tests to prevent or diagnose diseases early, such as mammograms and colonoscopies, or preventative treatments, such as aspirin to prevent heart attacks. While many are fearful of "bad news," and therefore forego any screening tests, isn't it better to make decisions based on knowledge and information, as opposed to burying one's head in the sand? If we never take our temperature, do we never have a fever? Currently, early diagnosis and treatment is our best tool in the battle against cancer. While our hope is to prevent cancer entirely, this is not the present environment. We must identify cancer early and eradicate it. Delayed diagnosis not only changes survival rates, but it dramatically increases the cost of diagnosis and treatment [22].

Tertiary prevention focuses on patients with chronic diseases, such as COPD (chronic obstructive pulmonary disease), diabetes, and hypertension. The aim is to either prevent worsening of the condition, minimizing exacerbations, or preventing complications associated with poor treatment control. Most patients diagnosed with diabetes or hypertension have difficulty in accepting treatment, because they have no symptoms. Why take medication, change dietary habits, and change behaviors, when we feel good? This is where the relationship between provider and patient is so important. In order to transform healthcare, patients must trust their provider's recommendations, and providers must educate their patients appropriately, so that the common goal of health has shared responsibility [22].

Individual responsibility as a patient must exist for success in the (proposed) transformed healthcare milieu. The adage "An ounce of prevention is worth a pound of cure" is appropriate for this discussion. The success of preventive health measures depends upon an informed provider, as well as a willing patient. However, the downstream results of such efforts will surely lead to decreased cost and a healthier society. There also must be consequences for those who refuse to comply. Our current laws place the sole responsibility on the provider to ensure that the patient is adherent with medications or treatment recommendations, and, if an adverse outcome ensues, the provider has legal liability, regardless of whether the patient was the cause of the complication. We will need to create a penalty system for those who consciously are noncompliant, and a benefit system for those who do.

A third component of patient accountability is recognition and acceptance of the limits of the healthcare system. This can take many forms: from the patient with a chronic illness who needs to recognize that the illness needs to be managed, and will not be cured; to the family of an elderly patient with a terminal condition; to the patient with chronic pain who needs to change their perspective and adjust to their physical limitations, rather than chasing a cure with surgery or medications. There are many other examples of unrealistic expectations that need to be muted. Our current payment system encourages providers to continue to treat, to provide false hope, to attempt procedures or surgeries that carry minimal or no chance of cure, but are handsomely compensated. Patient education, knowledge, and an understanding of disease are cornerstones for the development of an appropriate relationship between patient and provider, establishing trust and advocacy.

In order to achieve a healthy population, there are three responsible parties. Party number one is a Primary Care Provider (PCP) who is a patient advocate, a health counsellor, a manager of preventive screenings, a diagnostician, and a provider of treatment for common conditions. This provider should also know when specialty services are required by the patient. Party number two is an informed patient, educated to the nature of his or her condition(s), who understands the importance of healthy lifestyle choices, who has developed a relationship with a PCP, who tries to adhere to recommendations and is motivated to remain in good health. Party number three is a society which is willing to break down barriers to healthy living. This may relate to food deserts causing dietary inadequacies, housing issues, behavioral health and addiction treatment, cost of medications, and access to care. While these issues are commonly referred to as Social Determinants of Health, they are a vital part of healthcare. In the late twentieth century, Medicare would not pay for influenza vaccines; it was the patient's responsibility. However, they would pay for a patient's hospitalization due to complications of influenza infection. Eventually, rational thinking changed this paradoxical thinking. Why are the social determinants of health any different? Patients without access to healthy food will develop illnesses requiring significant monetary outlays. Why not pay for the correct prevention? Why not pay for addiction treatment, rather than pay for policing, arrests, jail, as well as healthcare costs?

If we believe that the health of a population includes ALL members of that population, as a society we must be prepared to provide services to those in need. Population health should not discriminate on the basis of insurance, race, citizenship, or wealth. Currently, the EMTALA law prohibits a healthcare facility from refusing emergency care for any reason. "In 1986, Congress enacted the Emergency Medical Treatment and Labor Act (EMTALA) to ensure public access to emergency services regardless of the ability to pay. Section 1867 of the Social Security Act imposes specific obligations on Medicare-participating hospitals that offer emergency services to provide a medical screening examination when a request is made for examination or treatment for an emergency medical condition, including active labor, regardless of an individual's ability to pay" [1]. Therefore, many uninsured or underinsured people use the hospital emergency room as their primary provider of medical services. It is much more efficient and cost-conscious to provide care in a PCP office, prevent complications, minimize preventable hospitalizations, and provide adequate social services to those in need, rather than shifting the cost of uncompensated emergency care and hospitalizations to the bills of patients with health insurance. This requires an honest assessment of health care costs and a desire by our society to acknowledge those in need, and a willingness to help [23]. As a society, we must agree that our goal is to create a healthier society, not just a healthier few. Change can not occur, unless the majority believes that such change is for the better. This means the betterment of all.

# 7

# Changing Behaviors

Having already discussed patients becoming active participants in their health journey, it is appropriate to view other areas of change required for success. Physician education has not changed dramatically in the last 50–75 years. Some information has changed, with new diagnostics, treatments, and medications. In addition, the manner of education is changing, with a focus on systems in health and disease. Previously, medical students would struggle to learn anatomy, physiology, pathology, and pathophysiology in separate courses. Nowadays, most schools teach all four areas of health and disease as they pertain to specific organ systems. This method is enhanced by practical problems in a case study, relating the book knowledge to a specific patient experience. Once the students graduate and begin their clinical training, they learn how to perform procedures, diagnose and treat disease, interpret diagnostics, and care for sick patients. Very little if any training is spent on the prevention of disease. Doctors in residency (training) spend the majority of their time in the hospital setting, learning from and caring for sick patients. This is because our entire healthcare system is focused on treatment of disease, from an educational level, an expense level, a compensation level, and a patient level. The perception is that the value of our healthcare system only exists when there is sickness and disease. This perception encompasses patients, providers, health plans, hospitals, government, and all ancillary business associated with the healthcare system, such as pharma and medical device manufacturers, among others.

When looking at the compensation associated with the various medical specialties, the highest salaries are in the surgical fields, oncology, and procedure oriented medical fields. If a physician could prevent a patient

*Transforming Healthcare: An Insider's Look on Why and How*, First Edition. Morey Menacker.
© 2022 John Wiley & Sons, Inc. Published 2022 by John Wiley & Sons, Inc.
Companion website: www.wiley.com/go/menacker/transforminghealthcare

from requiring surgery, shouldn't that be worth at least as much as the performance of the operation? If a physician could prevent a cancer, or identify it when a simple procedure would be curative, shouldn't the value of that service be at least equal to that of providing chemotherapy or radiation treatment? If we agree that there must be incentives in place in order to change behaviors, shouldn't those incentives align with maintaining health? If we provide the appropriate incentives to physicians in order for them to focus on health as opposed to disease, it is a natural step that medical training will follow suit and focus on health. If training programs focused on health while physicians were still compensated for treating disease, our trainees would revolt. They would continue to focus their energy on whatever incentives were driving the active medical community.

Starting in the Middle Ages, and persisting through the eighteenth century, bloodletting was an accepted method of treating illness. There were very few treatments or remedies for disease, and it was believed that by removing blood, the "bad humours" would be eliminated. Bloodletting was a treatment for any and all illnesses. Today, our equivalent to bloodletting is pharmaceuticals. We need pills to lose weight, pills to gain weight, pills to increase appetite, and pills to decrease appetite. If we want something to go away, we need a pill. If we want something to happen, we need a pill. If we want something to shrink we take a pill. If we want something to grow, we take a pill.

The over-reliance on medication has been driven by marketing on the part of the pharmaceutical industry. It has been warmly received by the medical community, because the perception is that there is a pill for everything, and the doctor just has to prescribe the right one. Patients are brainwashed into thinking that they require a prescription every time they see the doctor, and doctors are willing and able to comply. The perception allows physicians to avoid difficult discussions, explanations of symptoms, education about health, and avoidance of the ignominy of not knowing. Polypharmacy is an unspoken epidemic in this country. Medication interactions, toxicities, and side effects are major drivers of cost, morbidity, and even mortality. If providers are trained how to level set patient expectations, to educate patients, to utilize nonpharmacologic treatments, and to consider complementary medicine treatments, we can begin to wean our dependence on medication. The pharmaceutical industry has changed the way we can treat illness and has been a driver in increasing longevity. However, as part of our transition from sick care to healthcare, we must recognize that more medicine is not always better medicine.

Another area where behavior change is needed is the acceptance of the fact that life itself is a terminal condition. Everyone who lives must eventually die. Our goal is to make life as long as possible and as healthy as possible. The question arises about prolonging life. As a country we spend exorbitant amounts on the final year of life. The question here is not whether we spend money, but whether we are doing the right thing for the patient. Most patients with terminal cancer continue to receive chemotherapy even after it is clear that recovery is not possible. We cannot expect the patient to be able to make such a significant decision without appropriate knowledge, counseling, and advocating on their behalf. Our oncologists are trained to treat cancer, not to discuss end of life care. However, they should be experts in end of life care. We cannot blame them; we must change the education they receive, the incentive they reach for, and the goal of providing what is best for the patient.

This discussion leads to the issue of long-term care or nursing home care. A significant number of elderly patients cannot care for themselves and have no family members willing or able to care for them in the home setting. These patients spend their final days (years) in a facility. Medical services for these patients are paid for by Medicare, but the daily fee is not a covered expense. This must be paid for by the individual or by a health plan, if the patient has long-term care insurance. Most patients spend all of their savings on nursing home costs, and then must apply for Medicaid, which pays for long-term care. Many nursing home residents suffer from dementia, and worsen because of the unfamiliar surroundings, the isolation, and complications of inactivity. Routinely, these patients are hospitalized and then return to the same facility for a subacute care (a subacute nursing facility, SNF), which is paid for by Medicare (at a much higher rate than Medicaid), until their status is changed to long-term care again. While there is a need for some amount of institutional services for some elderly, the majority of patients would be better served to age in place, with their families, with home care to support their needs. This suggestion is much less costly and much more humane than the nursing home. In addition, if a frank and honest discussion is made with patient and family, hospitalization at the terminal stage of life is unwanted and unnecessary. Palliative care and hospice are the terminologies used in the medical profession for this service. It means the care of a patient to provide relief of symptoms and discomfort. This change in behavior requires education of all parties, an adjustment in covered benefits, and a willingness to have a frank discussion about what is life, what is death, and what is existence [24].

The discussion above is not suggestive nor supportive of rationing or limiting care in any way. The argument is that by spending on prevention of disease, by supporting healthy living, by caring for those in need, we can decrease the current expenditures toward healthcare. The incentive must be toward health. We will continue to treat disease, continue to explore new treatments, continue to care for our young and our old, and continue to provide the highest quality care in the world. The difference is that this quality care will be available to all and, hopefully, less of us will require it because we are healthy!

# 8

# Moving the Needle

In our current healthcare environment, there is a clear expectation of how much will be spent annually on patients with chronic illnesses. Every health insurance company, including CMS, our governmental health insurer, maintains actuarial tables in order to predict annual spend, and thereby setting premium cost. Medicare does not collect premiums, but does have to set an annual budget, as well as distribute capitated payments to Medicare Advantage health plans. These predictions are based on historical data and risk factor analysis – including demographics, age, sex, and zip codes. The zip codes have two purposes: the cost of care varies in different areas of the country, and also certain zip codes indicate economic status – which clearly affects prognosis (in our current system).

As we transform our care delivery system, it is obvious that we need to eliminate the current economic barriers to health. Social barriers need to be addressed as well, but this factor is more related to individualizing care based upon the patient's environment as well as their disease. If payment was tied to outcomes, then all insured patients should be treated equally. If everyone had insurance (access to care), then all economic barriers would vanish.

By using historical data (and coding) to determine the future cost of care, it follows that current healthcare financing does not anticipate any change in outcomes. Besides the reality that new treatments are becoming available regularly, there is no consideration of "changing the trajectory" of a chronic illness. When looking at chronic illnesses longitudinally, we see significant variability in treatment, utilization of services, spend, resources, and ultimately outcomes. This variability can

*Transforming Healthcare: An Insider's Look on Why and How*, First Edition. Morey Menacker.
© 2022 John Wiley & Sons, Inc. Published 2022 by John Wiley & Sons, Inc.
Companion website: www.wiley.com/go/menacker/transforminghealthcare

be related to the treatment recommended by the provider, the skill of the provider, the understanding of the natural history of the disease (by patient and/or provider), the ability to alter risk factors, and, most importantly – compliance.

In 2012, the Hackensack Alliance Accountable Care Organization (ACO) performed a study using congestive heart failure (CHF) patients who were frequently admitted to the hospital for exacerbations of CHF. These patients all had quality providers in both Cardiology and Primary Care, yet had frequent hospitalizations due to the severity of their heart disease. The ACO partnered with an analytics company and provided half of the patients with electronic tablets that had an embedded medication minder application. The tablet would alert the patient that it was time to take their medication and, if not addressed, would alert an ACO nurse. In addition, the tablet had patient education material available, with FAQ's. The incidence in hospitalizations dropped dramatically in the group with the tablets, while the control group had no change in their hospitalization rate. No changes were made to the care of the patient by the ACO, other than supplying the tablet, and calling the patient if they missed doses of medication regularly [25].

By no means am I suggesting that poor compliance is intentional. The most informed and focused patient would have difficulty being compliant, given the polypharmacy, the confusing orders: take twice a day vs. take every 12 hours, and the need to adjust medication based on their daily schedule. For example, no patient will take a diuretic, a water pill, prior to going out shopping or to a doctor's office. They were told to take it twice a day, so just take one at lunch and one at dinner: can't take it too late or sleep will be interrupted by bathroom breaks. It is the responsibility of the provider to understand the patient's limitations, and needs, and attempt to adjust the treatment to optimize compliance. However, in today's transactional environment, there is no time for that, nor any relationship built between patient and provider.

The above study, while only involving 50 patients, exemplifies that compliance to therapy is a dramatic driver of improved outcomes. In addition, the use of technology to ensure compliance is readily available, as these medication applications are widely available for smart phones. Therefore, by using technology to drive compliance, we can dramatically shift the trajectory of the patient's chronic illness. This will translate into a significantly decreased cost of care, subsidizing expanded insurance access, social services, and behavioral health. This, in turn, further minimizes the divergent health outcomes currently seen, based on economic status.

In general, there are many ways to alter the trajectory of a given chronic disease. Treatment variability is a major determinant in less than optimal outcomes. While there may be many different treatments available for a specific disease process, the choice of the best treatment depends upon the gathering of all information, analysis of the current literature, and including "social determinants" in the decision process. Once again, technology exists to make this a simple provider function. However, our electronic medical record systems don't talk to one another, and most providers use the EMR as a glorified word processing program, thereby eliminating the availability of data points to drive decision making. If outcomes were the driver of compensation, then providers would have an incentive to make the best treatment decision based on the information available, rather than relying on inadequate data and treatment plans learnt in medical training. Diagnostic tests would only be ordered when the result changes the treatment plan and are not based on the payment associated with the test.

While changes to the financing of healthcare will improve the overall health of our population, and also limit the persistent rise in the "cost of care," it will not resolve the socioeconomic, racial, and ethnic disparities in our country. These recommendations are not a panacea for all that is wrong, but, hopefully, will allow all Americans to have the same opportunity to live a healthy life with quality medical care.

## 9

# How Do We Pay for This?

A common argument for and against transforming our healthcare system is financing. Currently, a significant portion of the spending for healthcare is borne by private industry, in the form of employer-sponsored health insurance. The employee benefit is not considered as taxable earnings and the corporate spend is in pretax dollars. Many are fearful that a transformation would not only rid them of "choice," but would take away a significant financial benefit provided by their employer. The federal and state governments provide the majority of healthcare financing in the form of Medicare, Medicaid, and other government-funded payments. While the Congressional Budget Office purports that the administrative costs of the Medicare/Medicaid programs are less than private insurance companies, history tells us that the federal government is not an efficient spender. It is much more likely that the federal government utilizes "voodoo" accounting to minimize the actual administrative costs associated with managing CMS. Regardless of whether the federal government runs its health insurance business more efficiently than private health plans, the issue at hand is to provide the best healthcare possible to the entire country, and to use the financing system to drive quality and efficiency. This is not a discussion advocating a single or multiple payer system. The focus is to provide the best care to all and to utilize currently available dollars to support the health of our society.

There is a significant uninsured and underinsured population that does not receive routine preventive medical care, nor has a primary care provider to manage their medical problems. These individuals utilize hospitals and emergency rooms as their provider of choice. This is clearly not a cost-effective method of providing healthcare. First of all, symptomatic intervention and emergent treatment is not efficient or economical. Second, while the cost of care in an outpatient hospital setting is not transparent, the charges associated with such care are significantly higher than outpatient care in a clinic or physician's office. In addition, most of the bills generated from these services go unpaid. In order to maintain financial stability, hospitals then charge private insurance companies excessive fees, also known as cost shifting, in order to cover expenses. Therefore, all of the patients without health insurance are actually receiving overly expensive care, just because they do not have insurance! This care, while not paid for directly, is indirectly being subsidized by the insurance payments made for the care of the commercially insured patient. So, in essence, we are already paying for the care of the uninsured and underinsured. However, we are not efficient nor prudent in our spending.

The largest portion of the healthcare dollar goes toward hospital services. It is true that in the past 70 years, new treatments and technologies have changed the outcomes of many patients who otherwise would not have survived their illnesses. However, at what cost? Hospitals purchase the most up to date and expensive technology, not only to provide the best care, but to compete against other hospitals for patients. They need a continuous flow of patients to ensure a continuous flow of dollars. Most hospitals have budgets that ignore the actual cost of their work (cost-based accounting), but are only concerned about what they get paid for the procedure/diagnosis (accrual-based accounting). Medicare and some private insurance companies utilize a DRG payment for hospital services. Therefore, hospitals are paid a flat rate for a hospital stay, based upon the accepted diagnosis that caused the hospitalization. Thus, if a patient is hospitalized with pneumonia, the hospital is paid a flat rate, whether the stay is for three days or six days. This concept was developed and implemented in order to limit unnecessary procedures, as the payment will not change. However, a tactic used by many hospitals to shorten hospitalization is to discharge patients to a nursing facility who are not prepared to go home. The moniker attached to these locations is a Subacute Nursing Facility, or SNF. These facilities often are linked to hospital corporations, and charge daily rates to Medicare. That way, the hospital can fill the bed with another Diagnosis Related Group (DRG) payment, and also get paid for the patient in the nursing facility. A single payment for acute and post-acute care would eliminate

20–40% of all admissions to these nursing facilities. Payment to acute and post-acute care facilities, combined, costs about 60 cents of every healthcare dollar [26].

If you asked a hospital finance expert what the real cost of providing care for a patient requiring gall bladder surgery – a common occurrence in every hospital – they could tell you what they charge, what they get paid, but not what the cost was. Other than the Federal and State governments, hospital budgets are the only organizations that can ignore cost.

In many urban and suburban locales, hospitals compete against one another for patients. This is not primarily related to a desire to care for the most patients, but a need to perform as many procedures as possible, in order to get a return on investment from their expensive technology purchases. The converse is true in our rural communities. It is so costly to run a hospital, that many small hospitals in rural areas are forced to close. Dollars are being wasted in high population density areas on "competitiveness," while our low density areas are losing access to care. How do we resolve this conundrum?

Part of the solution lies in changing our current standard payment model. Our payment model compensates providers based on procedures performed, not outcomes. The more sophisticated the technology, the higher the compensation. Appropriate utilization is the responsibility of the insurance plan. While there may be an "appropriate" indication for the procedure, its effect upon the patient's outcome is not considered. Robots are now frequently used to assist and even perform surgeries. While the value of a robot performing a procedure that requires ultimate precision is obvious, these robots are being used to assist in appendix and gallbladder surgery, where microscopic precision is not a priority. Robotic surgical support is not a necessity, does not improve surgical outcome, and lengthens the procedure. Not only does this increase the cost, due to increased operating room time, but risk to the patient is significantly increased due to prolonged anesthesia. Then why the use of robots? The payment for robotic surgery far surpasses the payment for standard surgery.

If utilization was made the responsibility of the provider of services, would there be a decrease in costly diagnostics and therapeutics? In addition to technology, providers are currently compensated purely on their volume of work, no matter the outcome. Theoretically, a surgeon could be compensated for a hernia repair, and then be compensated again and again for repairing the same recurrent hernia, all on the same patient, even though he performed all the surgeries. Not that any physician would intentionally proceed in this fashion, but clearly the current payment and outcome goals are not aligned.

Our entire healthcare payment system is designed to compensate for treating the sick, not keeping people healthy. Rather than calling this book "Transforming Healthcare," perhaps it should be called "Transforming Sickcare (into Healthcare)."

All health insurance companies (including CMS) have a calculated anticipated annual healthcare spend for every insured person in the United States. This is how premiums are determined, Medicare is budgeted, and Medicare Advantage plans are funded. If we assigned large groups of people to specific healthcare delivery systems and provided global funding to these systems, then the responsibility for care, as well as the responsibility to control spending, would become the provider of care's concern and responsibility. This would align outcomes, utilization, and finance. These healthcare systems could be self-sufficient, providing primary and specialty care, as well as inpatient and outpatient services. Alternatively, they could also be hospital systems that purchase outpatient care services or outpatient organizations that purchase hospital services. Essentially, the assigned organization would purchase whatever services were not owned or leased, based upon contracted rates. The healthier the population becomes, the less the expense and the more money for the healthcare system. Stop-loss insurance coverage could be used by organizations tepid to take full risk. This involves an organization sharing excessive financial risk with a secondary insurance provider, for an annual premium. This also alleviates concerns for outliers and exorbitant costs. Rural locations could be aligned under the auspices of a regional healthcare system, with a focus on local patient stabilization (urgent care/icu) and transport to the regional hospital when needed. Investment in a transportation infrastructure, such as helicopters, would yield significant returns in health outcomes.

This proposal is a system for provision of healthcare services to all within our country. This type of system is feasible in a single payer model, or in a multiple payer model, as long as all individuals have insurance provided. Whoever acts as insurance intermediary, whether a public or private entity, will be responsible for appropriate global payment for patient panel size and severity of illness. They must also maintain records documenting diagnoses, outcomes, and efficiencies. As far as individual payment to providers is concerned, this would be the responsibility of the healthcare organization. Whether the organization chooses to employ providers, pay on a fee schedule, or create a partnership organization is dependent on the organization and its relationship with the local providers.

In addition, this model would drive competing hospitals to work together, decrease the technology wars, share resources, and purchase services from each other. Providers could remain independent, if desired, and sell their services to any system. The priority for all would be improved outcomes and the health of the population. Improving a population's health would take on many forms. Housing may be supplied, if needed. Nutritional needs would be prioritized. Elimination of obstacles to health maintenance would be the objective for the health system, for improvement, and amelioration. If the provider of care holds the purse strings, that organization may decide to invest in social services and programs that have been shown to decrease illness, noncompliance, and chronic disease exacerbation, and therefore decrease the overall cost to the organization.

An example of the improvement possible would be the patient with frequent hospitalizations for alcohol abuse. The healthcare organization could seek a more cost effective method of treating the patient, as in alcohol rehabilitation, and align the treatment with psychotherapy to identify a trigger for the aberrant behavior. It is in the interest of the organization to improve the health of the patient, as his health costs are tied to their bottom line. Instead of trying to instill a humanistic philosophy upon our entire population, in order to create the empathy required to change the plight of our underserved, this concept encourages the provision of care to the tired, poor, huddled masses, by aligning financial success with the health of an entire population. While a humanistic philosophy is an enlightening aspiration for us all, we physicians must deal with reality.

There are many opinions and recommendations as to how healthcare should be transformed in order to provide care to all without global bankruptcy. The model suggested, while less obtrusive than most alternatives, still requires significant support from all parties involved, and requires a major behavior change from providers and patients. The task is large, but the status quo is unsustainable.

# References

1 CMS.gov. (2021). 'CMS' program history.
2 Gordon, J.S. (2021). *A short history of American Medical Insurance.* Imprimis.hillsdale.edu.
3 Mayes, R. (2006). The origins, development, and passage of Medicare's Revolutionary Prospective Payment System. *Journal of the History of Medicine and Allied Sciences*, 10, 1093.
4 McCormack, L. and Burge, R. (1994). Diffusion of medicare's RBRVS and related physician payment policies. *Health Care Financing Review.*
5 AMA-assn.org. (2021). RBRVS overview.
6 Wikipedia.org. (2021). Resource-based relative value scale.
7 Kurani, N., McDermott, D., and Shanosky, N. (2020). *How Does the Quality of the U.S. Healthcare System Compare to Other Countries?* Healthsystemtracker.org.
8 Schutte, S., Acevedo, P., and Flahault, A. (2018). Health systems around the world – a comparison of existing health system rankings. *Journal of Global Health.*
9 Britannica.com. (2021). Public Health-National developments in the 18th and 19th centuries.
10 CDC.gov/MMWR. (1999).Ten great public health achievements – United States, 1900–1999.
11 Merriam-Webster.com. (2021). Healthcare.
12 HHS.gov (2019). About the affordable care act.
13 Mcguire, T., Newhouse, J., and Sinaiko, A. (2011). An economic history of medicare part C. *The Milbank Quarterly.*
14 Fernandez, V. (2017). Ins and outs of HCC's. *Journal of AHIMA.*

*Transforming Healthcare: An Insider's Look on Why and How,* First Edition. Morey Menacker.
© 2022 John Wiley & Sons, Inc. Published 2022 by John Wiley & Sons, Inc.
Companion website: www.wiley.com/go/menacker/transforminghealthcare

**15** DuGoff, E. and Chao, S. (2019). What's driving high disenrollment in Medicare advantage? *Inquiry.*

**16** Bodenheimer, T. and Sinsky, C. (2014). From triple to quadruple aim: Care of the patient requires care of the provider. *Annals of Family Medicine.*

**17** Lewis, N. (2014). *A Primer on Defining The Triple Aim.* IHI.org.

**18** Hopkinsmedine.org/news. (2016). Study suggests medical errors now third leading cause of death in the U.S.

**19** Bruenig, M. (2019). *Health Insurance Churn is A Nightmare.* Peoplespolicyproject.org.

**20** Bruenig, M. (2019). *People Lose their Employer-Sponsored Insurance Constantly.* Peoplespolicyproject.org.

**21** Google.com. (2021). Inertia.

**22** IWH.on.ca. (2015). Primary, secondary, and tertiary prevention.

**23** CMS.gov. (2021). Emergency Medical Treatment & Labor Act.

**24** ASPE.hhs.gov (1994). Subacute care: review of the literature.

**25** Riserbato, R. (2020). *The Plain-English Guide to Cost-Based Pricing.* Blog.hotspot.com.

**26** HIMMS.org/mobilehealthit (2014). Use case study: "Remote patient monitoring for chronic disease".

# Index

*Transforming Healthcare: An Insider's Look on Why and How*, First Edition. Morey Menacker.
© 2022 John Wiley & Sons, Inc. Published 2022 by John Wiley & Sons, Inc.
Companion website: www.wiley.com/go/menacker/transforminghealthcare